Nursing & Health Survival Guide

Palliative Care

Heather Campbell

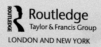

R Routledge
Taylor & Francis Group

LONDON AND NEW YORK

First published 2012 by Pearson Education Limited

Published 2014 by Routledge
2 Park Square, Milton Park, Abingdon, Oxon OX14 4RN
711 Third Avenue, New York, NY 10017, USA

Routledge is an imprint of the Taylor & Francis Group, an informa business

ISBN 13: 978-0-273-76062-7 (hbk)

British Library Cataloguing-in-Publication Data
A catalogue record for this book is available from the British Library

Library of Congress Cataloging-in-Publication Data
A catalog record for this book is available from the Library of Congress

Typeset in 8/9.5pt Helvetica by 35

Printed in the UK by Severn, Gloucester on responsibly sourced paper

contents

Palliative medicine and care aims to support individuals and their families with life-threatening and often life-limiting illness. This care is not new but it began as a formal discipline with the emergence in the UK of the modern hospice movement founded by Dame Cecily Saunders in the 1960s. Recognition of the speciality of palliative medicine happened in the 1980s. Since then the philosophy has been applied in a variety of settings, in a number of countries for a range of life-limiting conditions.

What is palliative care?

The term palliative is derived from the Latin verb *palliare* which means 'to cloak'.

Reference / Regnard, C.F.B. and Kindlen, M. (2002) *Supportive and Palliative Care in Cancer*. Abingdon: Radcliffe Medical Press.

The most widely recognised definition is that of the World Health Organization (WHO 2002) and examines the needs of the adult patient:

Palliative care is an approach that improves the quality of life of patients and their families facing the problems associated with life-threatening illness, through the prevention and relief of suffering by means of early identification and impeccable assessment and treatment of pain and other problems, physical, psychosocial and spiritual.

Palliative care:

- Provides relief from pain and other distressing symptoms
- Affirms life and regards dying as a normal process
- Intends neither to hasten nor postpone death
- Integrates the psychological and spiritual aspects of patient care
- Offers a support system to help patients live as actively as possible until death
- Offers a support system to help the family cope during the patient's illness and in their own bereavement
- Uses a team approach to address the needs of patients and their families, including bereavement counselling, if indicated
- Will enhance quality of life, and may also positively influence the course of illness
- Is applicable early in the course of illness, in conjunction with other therapies that are intended to prolong life, such as chemotherapy or radiation therapy, and includes those investigations needed to better understand and manage distressing clinical complications

Reference / http://www.who.int/cancer/palliative/definition/en/

■ WHEN DOES PALLIATIVE CARE BEGIN?

> **Reflection**
> Consider a situation where palliative care may be used for a patient who may not have a diagnosis of a life-limiting illness.

Support from the palliative care team may sometimes be needed for pain management postoperatively or to provide psychological support for patient and family in the event of a sudden unexpected death.

However, palliative care is part of the longer term support that should be offered to patients and families with life-limiting illness when care rather than cure is the emphasis:

- Supportive care
- End of life care
- Care in the last few days of life

They contribute to providing a seamless pathway and share the following characteristics:

- **E**nhancing quality of life
- **E**nabling autonomy and control in decisions
- **E**nsuring holistic care and symptom management

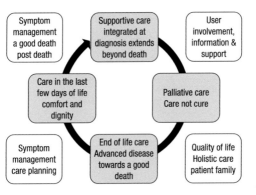

- **E**ncouraging a multidisciplinary approach
- **E**xtending to include family care

Summary
- Palliative care aims to improve quality of life when cure for a life-limiting condition is generally no longer an option
- It is part of a broader approach to care to support patient and family on their illness journey
- It includes care at the end of life and after death

'Palliative care is about putting life into a patient's days not days into their lives.'
Nairobi Hospice

■ NATIONAL POLICY

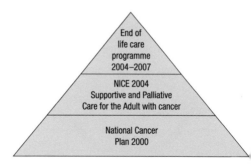

Key points
- Policy that has influenced palliative care initially started with cancer
- Policy identified the importance of patient choice
- Policy recommended the importance of integrated health and social care
- Policy recommended the use of systems and processes to optimise care

End of Life Care Strategy

The End of Life Care Strategy (Department of Health 2008) evolved from the End of Life Care programme. In summary it:

- Emphasised the importance of patient choice particularly around place of care at end of life
- Promoted the increased use of end of life care tools
- Recognised the need for all those with life-limiting illness to receive appropriate support and care
- Recognised the need to work towards enabling a good death

It anticipated that this could be achieved by developing an end of life care pathway with six key steps (see p. 6).

Reference / Department of Health (2008) *End of Life Care Strategy – Promoting high quality care for all adults at the end of life.* London: DH Publications.

Reflection
What do you notice about the steps of the pathway?

You may have noticed a number of things but the start of the pathway rests with having conversations about the future and the timing of these.

End of Life Care Strategy, DH 2008, with six key steps

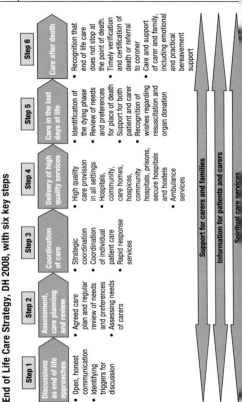

Step 1	Step 2	Step 3	Step 4	Step 5	Step 6
Discussions as end of life approaches	Assessment, care planning and review	Coordination of care	Delivery of high quality services	Care in the last days of life	Care after death
• Open, honest communication • Identifying triggers for discussion	• Agreed care plan and regular review of needs and preferences • Assessing needs of carers	• Strategic coordination • Coordination of individual patient care • Rapid response services	• High quality care provision in all settings • Hospitals, community, care homes, hospices, community hospitals, prisons, secure hospitals and hostels • Ambulance services	• Identification of the dying phase • Review of needs and preferences for place of death • Support for both patient and carer • Recognition of wishes regarding resuscitation and organ donation	• Recognition that end of life care does not stop at the point of death. • Timely verification and certification of death or referral to coroner • Care and support of carer and family, including emotional and practical bereavement support

Support for carers and families

Information for patients and carers

Spiritual care services

Determining end of life may not always be straightforward because each life-limiting condition has its own disease trajectory. A disease trajectory is a recognised general pattern of how certain life-limiting conditions progress over time. Some chronic conditions like end-stage heart failure and respiratory disease have acute episodes which are often interspersed with long periods of stability which mean that estimating when patients are at end of life may be more difficult.

The cancer trajectory, however, has been described as a steady progression but then a steep decline which usually ends in death and a point where end of life may be estimated.

> **Action**
> Read more about disease trajectories and prognostic indicators at www.goldstandardsframework.org.uk

■ WHO SHOULD RECEIVE PALLIATIVE CARE?

The WHO definition identifies that it should be patients and families with life-limiting illness. You will also have seen previously that it is cancer patients who receive palliative care most frequently. However, other patient groups who may need palliative and specialist palliative care include:

- Dementia
- Degenerative neurological conditions: Huntington's chorea, Parkinson's disease, multiple sclerosis (MS), motor neurone disease (MND)
- Organ failure including: renal, heart, respiratory and liver
- AIDS
- The older adult who is frail with multiple co-morbidities
- The younger adult with genetic conditions
- Children with life-limiting illness

■ WHO PROVIDES PALLIATIVE CARE?

Specialist palliative care services

Because palliative care is holistic care there are a number of disciplines to address the complexity of symptoms that may present. Specialist palliative care is usually delivered by experts in the area or who have specialist knowledge and skills.

Specialist palliative care team

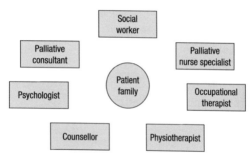

Most of this specialist care will be delivered in specialist inpatient units or hospices and hospitals or supporting community services in the patient's own home, care home or prison.

Generalist palliative care services

These include those who provide day-to-day care in the community or hospital setting:

- GPs
- Community nurses
- Health and social care registered and non-registered staff

Place of death all causes 2003

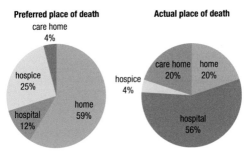

Preferred place of death

- care home 4%
- hospice 25%
- hospital 12%
- home 59%

Actual place of death

- care home 20%
- home 20%
- hospice 4%
- hospital 56%

Reflection

If palliative and end of life care can be delivered in a variety of settings why do you think a patient's preferred place of death is different from their actual place of death?

You might have identified the following:

- The patient may change their mind
- Patient choice may not be known
- The patient's condition may deteriorate in such a way that the preferred place of death is no longer seen as an option
- The nature of family support available
- Cultural and ethnic preference
- The nature of the life-limiting illness. For example, patients with non-solid tumours are more likely to have a hospital death
- Healthcare input available

See section on end of life care

Summary
- Policy has developed, particularly in the last decade, to address the specific needs of patient, family and carers at end of life
- Conditions other than cancer are seen as having palliative and end of life care needs, e.g. dementia, organ failure – heart, respiratory, renal, liver – degenerative neurological conditions
- A range of tools, processes and systems have been seen as facilitating care at the end of life. Liverpool Care Pathway, Supportive Care Pathway, Gold Standards Framework, Preferred Priorities of Care

*Palliative care is: 'To cure sometimes,
To relieve often, To comfort always'*
Dr. Robert Twycross

The patient journey

Points to consider

By the time a patient and their family are at the point of receiving palliative or end of life care:
- There may have been long periods of stability and wellness before they begin to deteriorate
- There may have been periods of active treatment with a real or perceived perception of cure
- Most life-limiting conditions will have had a serious impact on a patient's functional capacity, quality of life, relationships, aspirations and plans

Patient journey – key transition points and tasks

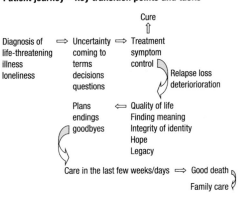

- The physical effects, impact of the disease and treatment may have diminished coping strategies and body responses
- The patient and family journey has often been described as a roller coaster

See section on a good death

Role of the nurse

There have been a number of studies that have looked at the role of the nurse in palliative care.

Reference / Davies, B. and Oberle, K. (1990) Dimensions of the supportive role of the nurse in palliative care. *Oncology Nursing Forum* 17: 87–94.

The Gold Standards Framework talks about the HEAD, HANDS and HEART of palliative care.

KNOWLEDGE	SKILLS	VALUES, BELIEFS
Clinical decision making	Maintaining comfort and dignity	Establishing rapport/connecting/letting go
Ethical decision making	Maintaining patient identity	Relationship building
Treatment options	Essential evidence-based care skills	Self-awareness
Pharmacology/pathophysiology	Touch	Emotional intelligence
Communication theory	Therapeutic touch	Empathy
Holistic assessment and symptom management	Communication skills	Helping to find meaning
Understanding boundaries/policies/systems		Restoring control/empowering
Creativity and innovation		Fostering hope
Advocacy/standing in the gap		Non-judgemental
Information giving/teaching		

Reflection

Consider whether you think there are any personal characteristics that are necessary for palliative care?

You might have considered the following and included more:

- Compassion
- Passion
- Warmth
- Self-awareness including coping strategies
- Confidence
- Self-belief
- Sense of humour
- Sense of worth

You may think that all of the above are important for any area of care but working regularly with patients and families with life-limiting illness may challenge our view of nursing and the world when dying is often so very present. Looking after ourselves is essential.

See section on self-care

Summary

- The patient journey is individualised and has often been described as a roller coaster for patient and family. However, there are shared elements including uncertainty, multiple losses, finding sense or meaning from life and dying, wanting quality of life, preparing for death, endings.
- The nurse in palliative care can support in this situation by restoring control, enabling the patient and family to prepare, maintaining integrity of identity, relieving distress and symptoms.

- The nurse requires a range of knowledge, skills and awareness of their own attitudes and beliefs.

  'You matter because you are you. You matter to the last moment of your life, and we will do all we can, not only to help you die peacefully, but also to live until you die.'
  Dame Cicely Saunders

Communication in palliative care

Effective communication is important in all areas of palliative and end of life care. Between multidisciplinary team (MDT), patient and family, within the MDT and other healthcare professionals, between patient and family.

Communication in palliative and end of life care is often associated with difficult conversations as well as the daily interactions and information giving.

Difficult conversations may include breaking bad news, discussing end of life care or responding to the distress of family, patient or colleague.

■ ESSENTIAL COMMUNICATION SKILLS

Use of non-verbal communication
- Lean forward
- Eye contact
- Relaxed posture – arms loosely on lap (don't slump!)
- Mirror the other person's position
- Relaxed but appropriate facial expression
- Nod head

Listening

- Pauses
- Silence
- Minimal prompts
- The 90-second monologue. Allow the patient/family member to speak uninterrupted with prompts only to elicit main concerns
- Acknowledging emotions: *I can see that you're . . .*
- Appropriate reassurance: *What you are feeling is quite natural . . .*
- Picking up cues
- Empathy – a desire to understand the client as fully as possible and to communicate this understanding
- Summarising
- Educated guesses – a guess based on past experience or previous knowledge used even when you may not have all the information required
- Acknowledging/reflection/paraphrasing
- Tone of voice
- Rate of speech

Information giving

- Tailored information (chunking and checking)
- Being jargon free!

Feedback and questioning

- Screening for underlying concerns
- Open questions
- Open directive questions
- Exploring

- Checking
- Clarifying
- Some closed questions
- Use something rather than anything – *Is there something else that you might wish to know?*

A simple way to remember?

Perceived facilitation skills for therapeutic communication (PEAS):

- **P**auses
- **E**mpathy
- **A**cknowledge
- **S**ummarise

■ BARRIERS TO COMMUNICATION

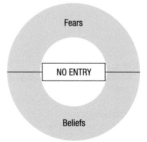

There are some well-established barriers to communication within this context.

Staff

FEARS	BELIEFS
• Unleashing strong emotions • Upsetting patients/ relatives • Patient refusing treatment • Difficult questions • Damaging the patient • Death anxiety	• Emotional problems are inevitable • Not my role • Talking raises expectations • Patient will fall apart • Will take too long
THE WORKING ENVIRONMENT	**SKILLS DEFICIT**
• No support or supervision • No referral pathway • Staff conflict • Lack of time	• In assessing knowledge and perceptions • Integrating medical and psychosocial modes of enquiry • Handling difficult reactions

References / Adapted from Wilkinson, S. et al. (1991) Factors which influence how nurses communicate with cancer patients. *Journal of Advanced Nursing* 16: 677–688, Maguire P. and Pitceathly C. (2002) Key communication skills and how to acquire them. *British Medical Journal* 325: 697–700.

These barriers may contribute to avoiding the patient's agenda. This may be demonstrated by:

• Inappropriate reassurance: *Don't worry, I'm sure it will be fine*
• Focusing on the physical issues, possibly those that you may be able to fix: *You say that you are not sleeping because thoughts go round and around in your head. I'll ask the doctor to see you and maybe a warm drink will help*

- Passing the buck (see above)
- Focusing on others: *You're obviously worried about your daughter. How is she managing?*
- Changing the subject

Reference / Adapted from Faulkner A. and Maguire P. (1994) *Talking to Cancer Patients and Their Relatives*. Oxford: Oxford University Press.

Reflection and action

What do you think your strengths and areas for development are in relation to communication skills? Undertake a SNOB analysis and identify one area where you might wish to make a commitment to change:

- **S**trengths
- **N**eeds
- **O**pportunities
- **B**arriers

■ THE SENSITIVE CONVERSATION – KEY CHARACTERISTICS OF COMMUNICATION

Having difficult, sensitive, distressing conversations require certain elements for progress to be made. These are likely to be:

- Having an existing relationship with the patient or family
- Maintaining trust
- Not lying
- Possessing effective communication skills and the confidence to use them
- Having the confidence not to use them – understanding boundaries and your own limitations
- Knowing who to refer on to

- Appreciating that there are no textbook responses
- Appreciating that the time and the place are not always within your control
- Respecting confidentiality

■ THE PROCESS – HINTS AND TIPS (PATIENT)

- **P**reparation. Information needed about the patient. Time, place, privacy. Am I the right person to do this?
- **A**genda. The patient's agenda – this may be eliciting what their understanding is; what their concerns may be; what is causing them distress; what their information needs are.
- **T**ime to talk. Use open questions to get the patient to talk (use why? judiciously) SILENCE. Remember the 90-second monologue.
- **I**nvolvement. Focus on what the patient is saying not on what you are going to say. Provide feedback, clarify, paraphrase and summarise.
- **E**motion. Acknowledge emotions and allow them to be ventilated.
- **N**ext steps. Provide information if required. Clarify expectations and what happens next.
- **T**elling the right people. Recording information.

■ BREAKING BAD NEWS

It is unlikely that as a student you will be put in the position of having to break bad news. This should be undertaken by senior personnel who have the right skills. However, bad news may mean different things to different people. It could mean that the patient may not go home because their transport has not arrived.

Models that can be used

BUCKMAN	KAYE
Setting	1. Preparation
Perception (patients)	2. What the patient knows
Invitation (to give knowledge)	3. What the patient wants to know
Knowledge (giving the information)	4. Giving a warning shot
Emotion	5. Allow denial
Strategy and summary	6. Explain if requested
	7. Listen to concerns
	8. Encourage ventilation of feelings
	9. Summarise
	10. Offer further information, support

References / Buckman R. (2010) *Practical Plans for Difficult Conversations in Medicine.* Baltimore: John Hopkins University Press; Kaye P. (1996) *Breaking Bad News: A Ten Step Approach.* Northampton: EPL Publications.

■ TOUCH

Touch can be powerful. Rousseau and Blackburn suggest that spontaneous touch may, at least at that particular moment, 'lessen the burden of disease' even when there is no available cure and therefore in itself could be seen as therapeutic. Think about it!

Reference / Rousseau P.C. and Blackburn G. (2008) The touch of empathy. *Journal of Palliative Medicine* 11(10): 1299–300.

■ WHAT HAPPENS IF?

These are suggestions only, there is no textbook answer

As a student nurse it is important to check fairly early on whether you have the 'authority' to become engaged in these types of conversations. Every clinical area differs. If the answer is yes, know your own limitations.

The patient asks me a difficult question, e.g. *Am I dying?*

1 Don't panic!
2 Sit at the patient's level. Use non-verbal communication skills (see section on the sensitive conversation) to demonstrate your willingness to engage
3 Give the impression you have time. Appear relaxed
4 Let the patient know that he/she is being heard. It may have taken much courage to ask the question
5 Do not give false reassurance (this is common) 'Of course you're not' 'Everybody's dying'

Reflection
Consider the following responses and your thoughts and feelings about them. What would work for you?

— *'I'm really sorry but I don't know. I'll get x to come and talk with you as soon as I can'*
— *'I'm really sorry but I don't know. I'll get x to come and talk with you as soon as I can but is there something I can do?'*
— *'That must have been a difficult question to ask'* (empathise). *'What makes you think you're dying?'* (an open ended question gives you time, gives you insight into the patient's understanding, enables you to correct misunderstanding if necessary)

— *'That must have been really difficult to ask. What is it that's worrying you?'*

The patient does not want me to tell his/her family that he/she has a life-limiting condition or the prognosis to be shared

If the patient has capacity then this has to be respected. However, it is important to discuss the value of sharing with his/her family. This might include putting financial affairs in order, preparing children, building bridges.

The family of a patient does not want me to give the patient bad news about his/her condition

Gently explain that if the patient asks then that information cannot be withheld from them. Explore the reasons for their concern about disclosure.

Summary
- Effective communication skills are essential in palliative care
- Work with the patient's agenda – establish what they already know and then how much they want to know
- Acronyms are useful but there are no set answers
- Respect confidentiality. Only share with the right people

'We will never meet everyone's expectations, but the skill and effort that we put into our clinical communication does make an indelible impression on our patients, their families, and their friends. If we do it badly, they may never forgive us; if we do it well, they may never forget us.'
Dr. Rob Buckman

Holistic assessment

■ **TOTAL PAIN**

Assessment of patients and families with life-limiting illness involves the nurse needing to understand how the disease process impacts on all areas of their lives. This notion of the holistic experience was termed by Cicely Saunders as 'total pain': 'total pain is the suffering that encompasses all of a person's physical, psychological, social, spiritual, and practical struggles'.

Reference / Richmond, C. (2005) Dame Cicely Saunders. *British Medical Journal* 33: 238.

Holistic assessment involves understanding the relationships between these elements and although they may be assessed separately they all contribute towards the whole experience and person.

Reflection

John is 46 years of age and has motor neurone disease. He has difficulty walking and has difficulties swallowing and talking. Previously a teacher, he has had to give up work and attends a day hospice once per week. He experiences muscle cramps and excessive drooling is an issue. His wife has just given up work to be his main carer. His two children are at senior school and the eldest is taking exams.

What might be the non-physical elements of his 'pain'?

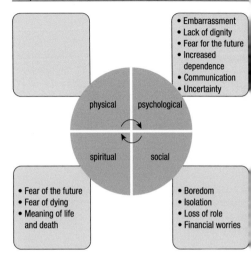

- Embarrassment
- Lack of dignity
- Fear for the future
- Increased dependence
- Communication
- Uncertainty

physical

psychological

spiritual

social

- Fear of the future
- Fear of dying
- Meaning of life and death

- Boredom
- Isolation
- Loss of role
- Financial worries

Factors that will influence the experience of life-limiting illness and total pain include:

- Age
- Gender
- Culture
- Religious views
- Personality
- Mood
- Previous life experiences
- Social support

- Perceived control
- Time to prepare
- Coping strategies

■ ASSESSMENT PROCESS

Assessment is an important process of care planning in any area of care. However, specific challenges may exist in palliative care:

- Complexity of symptoms
- Sensitive issues, e.g. dying, prognosis, treatment changes along the disease trajectory
- Barriers to communication in patient, family and self
- Ensuring continuity within a multiprofessional team

Skills required

- Communication skills (see section on communication in palliative care)
- Enabling therapeutic relationship (see section on communication in palliative care)
- Systematic questioning and processing
- Accurate recording
- Appropriate sharing

■ USING ASSESSMENT TOOLS

There are a number of issues to consider when assessing palliative and end of life needs. Bear in mind that the majority of assessment tools are not specific to palliative care, may not be culturally sensitive and when validated for palliative care have usually been researched with cancer patients.

Examples of assessment tools used in palliative care

DOCUMENT	TYPE	REFERENCE	COMMENT
PEPSI COLA	**Holistic assessment** **Physical** **Emotional** **Personal** **Social support** **Information and communication needs** **Control and information** **Out of hours** **Living with your illness** **Aftercare**	**Gold Standards Framework** www.goldstandardsframework.org.uk	Palliative specific. Could be used in a variety of settings but particularly useful for community care
FICA	**Spiritual assessment** **Faith** **Importance and influence** **Community** **Address or application**	Bourneman T., Ferrell B. and Puchalski C.M. (2010) Evaluation of the FICA tool for spiritual assessment. *Journal of Pain and Symptom Management* 40(2): 163–73.	Not palliative specific. Others include: SPIRIT Ambuel B. and Weissman D.E. (1999) Fast Fact and Concept 19: Taking a Spiritual History. End of Life Education Project http://www.eperc.mcw.edu/fastFact/ff_19.htm

DOCUMENT	TYPE	REFERENCE	COMMENT
PLISSIT	**Sexual assessment** **P**ermission (assessment) **L**imited **I**nformation (education) Specific **S**uggestion (counselling) **I**ntensive **T**herapy (referral)	Katz A. (2007) Sexual health assessment. In: Breaking the Silence on Cancer and Sexuality: A Handbook for Healthcare Providers. Pittsburgh, PA: Oncology Nursing Society, pp.19–29.	Not palliative specific Others include: **Pleasure** Schain W. (1988) cited in Mick J., Hughes M. and Cohen M.Z. (2004) Using the BETTER model to assess sexuality. *Clinical Journal of Oncology Nursing* 8: 84–86. **Alarm** Andersen B.L. (1990) How cancer affects sexual functioning. *Oncology* 4(6): 81–88. **Better** Mick J., Hughes M. and Cohen M.Z. (2004) Using the BETTER model to assess sexuality. Clinical *I Journal of Oncology Nursing* 8: 84–86.

Other tools
- Abbey Pain tool for individuals with cognitive impairment
- Wong–Baker Faces pain assessment tool for children or individuals with language barriers
- Distress/well-being thermometer

> **Action**
> Make a list of other assessment tools that you have used to assess patient/family needs at end of life

> **Summary**
> Assessment should:
> - Be holistic, integrating assessment tools as necessary
> - Adopt a team approach
> - Address sensitive issues

Symptom management

■ COMMON PHYSICAL SYMPTOMS

The symptoms below are often prevalent in advanced disease

- **Fatigue**
- Anorexia
- **Pain**
- **Dyspnoea**
- Cough
- Dry mouth
- **Constipation**
- Diarrhoea
- **Nausea and vomiting**
- Anxiety
- Low mood or depression

Those symptoms in bold have been identified as possibly the most prevalent in end of life care regardless of diagnosis.

Additional symptoms may occur as the disease progresses. This will impact on the way they are managed and may be indicators of advancing disease. Other symptoms that may present are:

- Oedema
- Lymphoedema
- Ascites
- Pleural effusion
- Itch
- Hiccups

There are some that develop at end of life or in the last few days of life and these will be addressed in the section on care in the last few weeks, days, hours.

Some symptoms, if not managed quickly, may shorten life and increase discomfort. These are often termed palliative emergencies and are discussed in the section on symptoms at the end of life.

■ PRINCIPLES OF SYMPTOM MANAGEMENT

- The emphasis is on palliation not cure
- Symptoms are multidimensional, therefore management should be achieved through a multiprofessional team approach
- Correct the correctable
- Keep treatment straightforward
- Use pharmacological and non-pharmacological approaches
- Drugs should be prescribed PRN as well as regular doses
- Side effects of treatment should be anticipated
- Work with the patient and family to elicit their perception
- Involve the patient in decision making
- Specialist palliative care services may need to be used

Pain management

■ DEFINITIONS

'Pain is whatever the experiencing person says it is, and exists whenever he says it does' Margo McCaffery.

Reference / McCaffery, M. and Beebe, A. (1999) *Pain: Clinical Manual for Nursing Practice*, 2nd edn. St. Louis, MO: Mosby.

In the section on holistic assessment the concept of total pain was discussed. This clearly demonstrates that pain is complex and not just a physical sensation. Acknowledging the individual nature of the pain experience forms the basis of the pain assessment process.

Pain may be described in a number of ways in palliative care:

DESCRIPTIONS OF PAIN	HOW IT PRESENTS
Chronic pain	Persistent and constant in nature
Acute	Transient, may come on quickly, may be severe
Intractable or refractory	Persistent pain that does not respond to treatment
Baseline	Persistent pain. The average intensity of which may be worked out over 24 hours
Incident	Pain that may come on as a result of an action or activity

DESCRIPTIONS OF PAIN	HOW IT PRESENTS
Breakthrough pain	Exacerbation of pain which may occur despite patients receiving regular medication. May present as incident pain, without any known cause or just before the next dose is expected. Sometimes called episodic pain

■ CAUSES

- Nerve pain
- Bone pain
- Soft tissue or visceral pain
- Referred pain
- Phantom pain

Pain is also sometimes categorised as neuropathic or nociceptive.

Nociceptive

Pain detected and experienced by specialist sensory nerves called nociceptors. This may be as a result of injury, irritation or damage to tissue.

- Somatic – muscle and skin
- Visceral – organ

Neuropathic

Injury or compression to peripheral or central nervous system.

■ ASSESSMENT

Use your senses! This can be a starting point before asking questions.

Eyes

Does the patient look in pain? Are they guarding (protecting) areas of their body through positioning?

Hearing

Moaning, groaning or other sounds of distress. What are patients telling you (see section on communication)?

Smell

Not so obvious but consider offensive smells from urine or wounds for example.

Touch

Hot? Cold? Painful to touch? Tense or swollen?

■ ASSESSMENT TOOLS AND QUESTIONS

There are a number of assessment tools that may assist in this process which may cut down time. This is particularly important with the breathless patient or when fatigue is an issue.

Visual analogue scale

Where would the patient rate their pain on this simple scale?

0 · 10

No pain   Severe pain

Useful questions to ask

- Where is your pain? You may wish to use a body chart
- How long does it last?
- When does the pain occur?
- Is it related to any activity?
- What helps it or makes it worse?
- How would you describe it?

Or use the PQRST model (see below).

PQRST

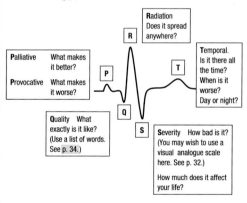

Palliative What makes it better?

Provocative What makes it worse?

Quality What exactly is it like? (Use a list of words. See p. 34.)

Radiation Does it spread anywhere?

Temporal. Is it there all the time? When is it worse? Day or night?

Severity How bad is it? (You may wish to use a visual analogue scale here. See p. 32.)

How much does it affect your life?

Reference / Adapted from Twycross R. (2003) *Introducing Palliative Care*, 4th edn. Abingdon: Radcliffe Medical Press.

Words that can be used to describe pain

Tingling (nerve)

Throbbing (may be bone, visceral)

Tight

Stabbing

Splitting

Burning

Colicky

Dull (may be bone, visceral)

Aching (may be bone)

Bruised

Tender

Shooting

Sharp (may be visceral)

Gnawing

Gripping

> **Reflection**
>
> Why might patients under-report pain?

You might have included:

- The need to experience pain
- Fear of being seen as a nuisance
- Stiff upper lip, not manly
- Cultural differences
- Fear that the disease may have progressed
- Fear of medications like morphine

■ MANAGEMENT

- Increasing pain may mean disease progression. This may be a reality or patient perception
- Pain may be a result of treatments or incidental illness, e.g. headache, arthritis
- There may be more than one pain present (see opposite)
- Not all patients with cancer have pain (approximately 25% may not have pain)

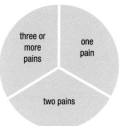

- Some patients may experience hyperalgesia (an increased sensitivity to pain) or allodynia (pain felt as a result of a stimulus that would not normally cause pain, e.g. light touch)

Glossary of terms

Adjuvent	Substance that enhances the effect of another drug Not usually used for analgesic purposes
Bioavaliability	The amount of drug that reaches its target site available once it has been absorbed and metabolised
Nerve block	An anaesthetic or anti-inflammatory injection that interrupts signals from a nerve or group of nerves (plexus) to manage pain

Naloxone	A drug that may be used to reverse the effects of opioid overdose if there is severe respiratory depression
Modified release	Medication that is used once pain is controlled and which has longer onset and longer duration, e.g. 12 hours
Opioid naive	Patient has not used opioids before
Standard or normal or immediate release products	Medication that has a quicker onset and a shorter duration, e.g. 4 hours
Titration	A process of incrementally increasing a patient's analgesia until pain relief is achieved

■ WHO PRINCIPLES

| | By clock | • Regular analgesia should be prescribed and administered at appropriate dose intervals
• Should also be given on time |
| | By mouth | • Preferred route of administration should be oral. However, disease progression may eventually mean that other routes would need to be considered |

	By ladder	• Provides principles of prescribing
		• Start on the bottom rung, i.e. with non-opioid
		• Progress on to opioids
		• Use adjuvant medications
		• There is no maximum dose for the top rung but specialist advice would be required
		• Particularly useful for visceral pain

Reference / World Health Organization (1996) WHO ladder. *Cancer Pain Relief*, 2nd edn. Geneva: World Health Organization.

Strong opioid ± Non-opioid ± adjuvents

STEP 3

Weak opioid ± adjuvent

STEP 2

Non-opioid ± adjuvents

STEP 1

MEDICATIONS USED

Always refer to *British National Formulary* (BNF) or *Palliative Care Formulary* (PCF) in the first instance.

	EXAMPLES	MAIN INDICATION	MAIN USE/DOSE RANGE	COMMENT
Non-opioid Paracetamol		Analgesic and antipyretic	Oral – tablet (500 mg–1 G) 4–6 hourly. Max dose 4 G in 24 hours) Rectal (suppository) 500 mg	Keep within recommended dose
Non-steroidal anti-inflammatory drugs	Ibuprofen	Inflammation Bone metasteses	Oral – tablet (200–400 mg tds/qds)	Caution with patients with peptic ulcer
	Naproxen		Oral – tablet (250–500 mg bd)	
	Diclofenac		Oral – tablet (up to 150 mg daily)	

	EXAMPLES	MAIN INDICATION	MAIN USE/DOSE RANGE	COMMENT
Weak opioids				
	Codeine	Mild to moderate pain	Oral – tablet (30–60 mg 4 hourly up to 240 mg in 24 hours)	Constipation
	Tramadol	Moderate to severe pain	Oral – tablet (50–100 mg 4 hourly. Max 400 mg in 24 hours)	Sometimes seen as a bridge between weak and strong opioids
	Co-codamol (codeine 30 mg/ paracetamol 500 mg)	Mild to moderate pain	Oral – tablet (2 tabs 4–6 hourly. Max 8 in 24 hours)	Codeine and paracetamol

	EXAMPLES	MAIN INDICATION	MAIN USE/DOSE RANGE	COMMENT
Strong opioids Morphine	Morphine	Severe pain (not that effective on its own with neuropathic or bone pain)	Oral – tablet (starting dose 5–10 mg) Oramorph oral solution (10 mg in 5 ml)	The drug of choice See below
	Diamorphine	Severe pain	Injection IM/SC (depends on previous opioid regime)	First line injectable Large amounts can be given in a small volume
Synthetic opioid	Fentanyl	Severe chronic pain which is being well managed	Transdermal patch (depends on previous opioid regime)	Available in 4 strengths Replaced every 72 hours

	EXAMPLES	MAIN INDICATION	MAIN USE/DOSE RANGE	COMMENT
	Alfentanil	Severe pain	Injection Spray/buccal or sublingual Syringe driver	Useful in patients with diminished renal function Short duration may be useful for incident pain
Semi-synthetic	Oxycodone	Severe pain	Oral normal (OxyNorm) or modified release (OxyContin) Immediate release as injection May be used in syringe driver	Used when morphine is not able to be used. Good bioavailability Approx 1.5 times more potent than morphine
Adjuvents Corticosteroids	Dexamethasone	Cerebral oedema Nerve compression	Oral	

	EXAMPLES	MAIN INDICATION	MAIN USE/DOSE RANGE	COMMENT
Muscle relaxant	Baclofen	Muscle spasm	Oral	Avoid sudden withdrawal
	Diazepam	Muscle spasm	Oral	
Anticonvulsant	Gabapentin Pregabalin	Neuropathic pain	Oral	Drowsiness Avoid sudden withdrawal
Antidepressant (tricyclic)	Amitryptyline	Neuropathic pain		Drowsiness Anticholinergic effects
Antispasmodics	Hyoscine butylbromide	Smooth muscle Spasm	Oral injection	
Bisphosphonates	Pamidronate	Bone pain	IV	
	Zoledronic acid		IV	

Action

Referring to BNF or PCF make further notes on side effects and other drugs not mentioned. Learn to recognise normal range of dosage.

■ MORPHINE

Points to be remembered:

- The first line choice, particularly for cancer pain
- Usually prescribed with a non-opioid
- Oral preparations are the first choice
- Available in normal or modified release
- Likely to cause drowsiness initially
- May cause a dry mouth – so attention to mouth care, use simple measures to relieve, see section on mouth care
- May cause nausea which usually passes but an antiemetic should be prescribed
- Will cause constipation, therefore an aperient to be prescribed
- If prescribed appropriately should not cause respiratory depression
- Other side effects include myoclonic jerks (involuntary twitches or jerks), dry mouth, sweating and hallucinations which may mean opioid toxicity and should be reported
- Does not cause psychological dependence when used as an analgesic in palliative care
- If toxicity suspected naloxone may be administered to reverse

Reflection

What concerns do you think patients and families may have when prescribed morphine or other opioids?

These may include:

- Fear of addiction
- Their condition is deteriorating and they are dying
- A form of euthanasia

Patients prescribed morphine for the first time may require careful explanation and support to understand its benefits and the reasons for using it.

■ OTHER WAYS TO MANAGE PAIN

- Educate your patient and families about their medications including side effects
- Enable concordance through education and finding ways to ensure that medications are taken regularly
- Complementary therapy
- Heat
- Cold
- TENS
- Palliative radiotherapy (for cancer)
- Positioning
- Pressure relieving/reducing aids
- Exploring distress and total pain
- Diversional activity
- Relaxation therapy
- Movement/rest
- Physiotherapy, particularly for patients who have muscle spasm, joint pain or diminished sensation in limbs

Nausea and vomiting

This is a common symptom in over half of patients with advanced cancer. The management of nausea and vomiting depends on the cause.

■ CAUSES

GASTROINTESTINAL	DRUGS	BIOCHEMICAL
<ul><li>Squashed stomach</li><li>Intestinal obstruction</li><li>Constipation</li><li>Gastritis</li><li>Delayed gastric emptying</li><li>Enlarged liver</li></ul>	<ul><li>Opioids</li><li>Palliative chemotherapy</li><li>NSAIDs</li><li>Steroids</li></ul>	<ul><li>Hypercalcaemia (high calcium)</li><li>Hyponatremia (low sodium)</li><li>Uraemia (high urea)</li></ul>
EAR	PSYCHOLOGICAL	CEREBRAL CORTEX
<ul><li>Middle ear infection</li><li>Vertigo</li><li>Labyrinthitis</li></ul>	<ul><li>Anxiety</li><li>Associations</li></ul>	<ul><li>Raised intracranial pressure</li><li>Sensitivity to sights and smells</li></ul>

■ ASSESSMENT

- Have patients lost weight?
- Are they dehydrated?
- What time of day is the vomiting happening? If it is in the morning it may be due to raised intracranial pressure
- Is it associated with eating? How soon after a meal?
- How much vomit is there? Large amounts may indicate gastric stasis
- What colour is it? Is there evidence of blood or 'coffee grounds'?
- Is vomiting preceded by retching or nausea?
- What helps vomiting or nausea?
- Is it prolonged, persistent nausea? May be metabolic or drug-induced
- Is nausea alleviated by eating?
- Is nausea associated with medications?

■ MANAGEMENT

Vomiting occurs when the vomiting reflex in the brain is stimulated by sensory messages from various parts of the brain and gastrointestinal tract. It in turn stimulates the vagus nerve and other cranial nerves to the stomach and upper gastrointestinal tract to cause vomiting to occur.

The importance of understanding the pathways and the neurotransmitters involved is important because:

1 The sensory pathways to the vomiting centre have different neurotransmitter receptor sites
2 Different antiemetics block different neurotransmitter receptors which in turn inhibit the sensory signals to the vomiting centre

General principles

- Treat the cause, e.g. constipation
- The antiemetic chosen depends on the cause. However, some are broad spectrum, e.g. cyclizine and levomepromazine. This means that they block a number of receptor sites.
- May need to be given via a parenteral route, e.g. syringe driver
- Some antiemetics should not be given together, e.g. cyclizine and metoclopramide

■ ANTIEMETICS

CAUSE	COMMONLY USED ANTIEMETIC
Drug-related Biochemical	Haloperidol
Cerebral cortex (intracranial pressure)	Dexamethasone
Ear (vestibular disturbance)	Cyclizine
Gastrointestinal	Metoclopramide or Cyclizine
Psychological	Diazepam

Other antiemetics

- Levomepromazine (broad spectrum)
- Ondansetron (not usually the first choice in palliative care but used with some chemotherapy regimes)
- Octreotide (reduces the volume of vomit)
- Hyoscine butylbromide (reduces the volume of vomit)

■ CARE AND SUPPORT

- Ask the patient to keep a record of vomiting episodes and nausea
- Regular mouth care
- Ice to suck if drinking makes the nausea/vomiting worse
- Small meals if food is tolerated. Little and often
- Avoid strong smells, e.g. wearing perfume, certain foods
- Complementary therapy, e.g. acupuncture or acupressure
- Reassurance that it may not last, e.g. when starting morphine or other opioids

Breathlessness

This is a distressing symptom which is common in a number of life-limiting conditions albeit for different reasons. It is often an indicator of a poor prognosis. For patients with chronic obstructive pulmonary disease (COPD) this may not necessarily be the case.

It is described by Twycross as the 'subjective experience of breathing discomfort' and may feature in 70% of patients in the last few weeks of life.

Reference / Twycross R. (2003) *Introducing Palliative Care*, 4th edn. Abingdon: Radcliffe Medical Press.

It is described by patients as:
- *'Part of the way toward choking'*
- *'Going to take your last breath'*
- *'Breathing through cotton wool'*
- *'Wishing you could get more breath, getting exhausted'*
- *'It frightened the life out of me, like a suffocation'*

- 'It feels like I'm not going to breathe again'
- 'Breathing while you're drinking a glass of water or have your mouth half full'

Reference / Corner, J., Plant, H. and Warner, L. (1995) Developing a nursing approach to managing dyspnoea in lung cancer. *International Journal of Palliative Nursing* 1: 5–11.

■ CAUSES

The causes of breathlessness are multifaceted and often related to the disease process and the individual's perception of feeling breathless:

- Cancer or the respiratory tract or pulmonary metastases
- Anaemia
- Pleural effusion
- Ascites
- Weakening respiratory muscles, e.g. MND
- Infection
- Chronic respiratory or heart disease
- Anxiety and fear

■ SUPPORT AND MANAGEMENT

It is suggested that general supportive measures are often effective in managing palliative breathlessness. The list below suggests ways in which breathlessness may be relieved:

- Helping the patient to find a position that helps. Sitting comfortably – sitting upright, or the orthopnoeic position
- Using a fan, particularly a hand-held one (stimulates branches of the trigeminal nerve)
- Adequate room ventilation
- Using closed questions
- Complementary therapy including aromatherapy

- Relaxation/distraction exercises
- Pacing one's activities
- Creating practical living arrangements, e.g. moving furniture
- Mechanical interventions, e.g. non-invasive positive pressure ventilation. May be used for patients with MND
- Breathing exercises (see below). Involve the physiotherapist

■ BREATHING EXERCISE

1 Sit with patient
2 Explain what you are going to do
3 Demonstrate the following
4 Relax shoulders – gently lower and relax the muscles
5 Concentrate on breathing
6 Take a short breath in
7 Place hand on tummy and breath out under your hand
8 Concentrate on breathing out slowly
9 Ask patient to try it
10 Ask them how they felt (closed questions)

■ PHARMACOLOGICAL MEASURES

Pharmacological measures will differ depending on the stage of illness and the cause of breathlessness they may include:

- Oxygen. In advanced cancer there is little evidence of its efficacy but may reduce anxiety. Usually 1–2 L/min
- Antibiotics
- Bronchodilators
- Steroids (usually with COPD)
- Oral morphine
- Midazolam or lorazepam

Constipation

Prevention is better than cure!

Disturbances to bowel function are common in palliative care. Constipation in particular because of:

- Use of opioids
- Reduced mobility
- Reduced appetite and fluid intake as the condition progresses
- Sweating (occurs with some cancers)
- Dehydration and fluid loss, e.g. vomiting
- Effects of disease, e.g. spinal cord compression, tumours of gastrointestinal tract, mouth, reduced nerve sensation in MS or cognitive impairment
- Biochemical – hypercalcaemia

Constipation can have serious effects on quality of life and can worsen other symptoms.

■ ASSESSMENT

- Your patient's normal bowel routine
- Your patient's mouth to rule out factors that inhibit eating and drinking. This includes thrush (yeasty smell, whitish creamy raised areas which if scraped leave areas that bleed, a burning sensation in mouth or throat), stomatitis (particularly if having chemotherapy). Mouth ulcers
- Issues around defaecation, e.g. pain
- Religious or cultural beliefs
- Your patient's toilet facilities. Perhaps they are not able to get to the toilet

■ MANAGEMENT

Laxatives

Prophylatic prescription of a laxative to be given regularly, doses may be higher than usual. If bowel obstruction suspected then further advice would be sought.

A stimulant with softening agent is often a starting point. A combined preparation reduces medication burden, e.g. co-danthramer, co-danthrusate. Refer to local clinical guidelines.

Fluids

Drink plenty. This may be difficult towards end of life when the patient may not be able to swallow, may feel sick or vomit, may be drowsy, may be fearful of urinary incontinence. Little and often, offering fruit juice rather than water if preferred.

Fibre

How realistic is this with diminished appetite, potential swallowing difficulties? Work with fruit juices, purées rather than high fibre cereal, breads etc. unless this is the patient's preference.

Exercise

Exercise or promote mobility. Not always an option.

Fatigue

Approximately 80% of patients with cancer, AIDS, heart failure, COPD and renal failure will experience fatigue.

Fatigue in advanced illness is reported to be unlike that experienced by the healthy person. Patients with life-limiting illness with fatigue describe it as:

- Being trapped in a failing body
- An energy drain
- A worse symptom than pain

Reference / Ream E. (2007) Fatigue in patients receiving palliative care. *Nursing Standard* 21: 49–56.

As a result they may have:

F Frustration – unable to function
A Attentional fatigue – lack of concentration
T Tolerance diminished – irritability
I Isolation
G Guilt
U Useless – a burden
E Emotional lability – depression

■ CAUSES

Fatigue may occur at any stage of the patient's journey. The causes are often interlinked.

- Anaemia
- Disease progression
- Sleep disturbance
- Reduced mobility
- Treatments

■ ASSESSMENT

Despite being so common it is often under-reported. Tools for evaluation include a simple visual analogue scale and the Brief Fatigue Inventory with a range of questions and visual analogue scales. However, simply raising the question with patients should provide permission for the patient to talk about it.

■ SUPPORT AND MANAGEMENT

This depends on the cause and stage of the patient's journey. Interventions include:

- Pacing activities. Energy conversation and expenditure. Saving energy for particular activities (e.g. going out) and then resting after
- Exercise. In palliative care this may not be that useful; however, to be encouraged if possible
- Distraction therapy
- Acupuncture and acupressure (seen to be useful in MS)
- Helping with sleep at the appropriate time of the day. Normal sleep patterns may be disrupted by dosing and resting
- Correcting anaemia and other physiological causes
- Investigating for hypercalcaemia
- Short-term use of steroids
- Psychostimulants (methylphenidate)
- Amantadine (in MS)
- Treatment of depression

Action
Read your local clinical guidelines and procedures for
further guidance

Summary
- The patient and family with life-limiting illness presents
  with many complex symptoms which will impact on their
  quality of life
- Some symptoms are more prevalent at certain times of
  a patient's journey
- Detailed, thorough, individualised assessment is
  essential
- Correct the correctable
- A holistic approach to management including
  pharmacological is essential
- Recognised standard management may not always be
  appropriate for patients at end of life

Care at the end of life

Some thought has been given to defining when a patient is at
end of life or dying. This has been primarily through the use
of prognostic indicators and the surprise question. Would you
be surprised if this patient was alive in 6 months – a year?

Reference / Gold Standards Framework (2010) GSF prognostic indicator
guidance. *End of Life Care* 4(1): 62.

This is not an exact science but it enables for
individualised care planning, choices and decisions.

■ SYSTEMS AND PROCESSES

Gold Standards Framework

An evidence-based approach to care for patients and families requiring palliative care. It emphasises the importance of co-ordination and organisation of care and has been applied in a variety of settings. It includes:

- **C**ommunication
- **C**o-ordination
- **C**ontrol of symptoms
- **C**ontinuity of care
- **C**ontinued learning
- **C**arer support
- **C**are of the dying pathway

Preferred Priorities of Care

A document that is now part of the NHS National End of Life Care programme. It provides opportunity and structure to discussing with a patient and family their wishes for care as their condition deteriorates. This might include preferred place of death.

Advance Care Planning

Advance Care Planning is a discussion between an individual and their carers that identifies:

- Wishes/values
- Concerns
- Preferences for care

to be respected and considered for a time in the future when the patient may no longer make or convey those decisions themselves.

It has two key components:

1 *Advance statements:* a discussion and record (optional) of a patient's and family's wishes and preferences for care. What a patient would like to happen.

2 *Advance decisions* (previously described as advance directives or living wills) to refuse treatment and life-sustaining treatment. What a patient would *not* like. This would include discussion around do not attempt resuscitation (DNAR) and other interventions. Because of the legally binding nature of advance decisions they should be documented and signed. Advance statements and decisions are taken into account when a patient no longer has **capacity**. While a patient has capacity care planning takes place on a regular basis with full involvement of patient (and family and carers).

Reference / NHS (2010) Advance Care Planning: A Guide for Health and Social Care Staff. www.endoflifecareforadults.nhs.uk

Lasting Power of Attorney (LPA)

LPA is a legal document that states in writing who can make decisions for a person if they *lack* capacity. It can relate to health and welfare or property and financial affairs.

> **Reflection**
> If you were to become seriously ill you would obviously have many concerns about your health but what other things would worry you as your illness progresses?

You might have considered the following. How will your family manage financially, where you want to die, funeral arrangements?

Symptoms at end of life

Many of the symptoms already addressed will begin or continue into the last few months of life although treatment will change. The aims of care, however, remain the same (see sections on what is palliative care and principles of symptom management). The patient's decisions about what treatment they would want, need to be considered in relation to the burden of treatment, the benefits versus risks and whether it would be futile to pursue a certain approach.

■ PALLIATIVE EMERGENCIES

In cancer particularly a number of situations may present that may seriously threaten life.
- Know your patient – history, treatment
- Your role is to recognise changes in your patient
- Report them immediately
- Support your patient with comfort measures, information

		COMPRESSION	OBSTRUCTION	
	Cytokines, parathormone-like hormones	Primary tumour of CNS, metasteses	Tumours in the chest, bronchus, vessels	Rare. Fungating wounds in neck or groin. Internal bleeding
Signs and symptoms	Nausea and vomiting, constipation, thirst and polyuria, drowsiness, confusion, eventual coma	Back pain often for some time, tingling, weakness, numbness Incontinence and perianal numbness are late symptoms	Breathlessness, headache Oedema of face and neck Dilated veins on chest wall	May be preceded by previous haemorrhage, bleeding Death often occurs in minutes
Treatment	Pamidronate infusion unless prognosis poor Rehydrate with IV fluids ? Treat cause	Urgent treatment to prevent paraplegia Dexamethasone Radiotherapy and surgery may be considered	Relief of acute symptoms Dexamethasone Reassurance ? Radiotherapy or chemotherapy to reduce tumour	Shout for help Stay with patient, have dark or red coloured towel Have someone to be with family Midazolam

Other complications include: bowel obstruction, fractures, epilepsy

■ DEPRESSION

This is an often overlooked symptom at end of life because of the natural sadness that will occur as end of life approaches.

Elisabeth Kubler Ross identified a number of stages that patients might progress through in preparation for death. One of which is depression.

1 Denial
2 Anger
3 Bargaining
4 **Depression**
5 Acceptance

Reference / Kubler Ross, E. (1997) *On Death and Dying*. Scribner: New York.

Reflection
How would you recognise depression in your patient?

This may be difficult as many of the symptoms that present with depression may occur as the result of the disease as well as adapting to dying.

■ ASSESSMENT

There are numerous assessment tools. Two of the simpler ones are:

- The distress thermometer, a vertical visual analogue scale where 0 is no distress and 10 is extreme distress.
- The screening question *'Are you depressed?'*

Reference / http://www.endoflifecareforadults.nhs.uk/tools/. . . / distress-thermometer

Your role

Know your patient: Ask questions:

- *How are things?*
- *How are you feeling today?*
- *What's been happening in the last week, etc?*
- *You don't seem yourself today. What's up?*

Report:

Life is just not worth living and other suicidal ideas.

■ SUPPORT AND MANAGEMENT

- Exploring worries or concerns is there anything practical that can be done?
- Relaxation and complementary therapy
- Recognising existential issues
- Therapies, e.g. CBT? Talking therapies
- Antidepressants: citalopram (SSRI – selective serotonin re-uptake inhibitors), mirtazapine

A good death

Preparing for end of life care requires numerous adjustments for patient and family. Cultural issues, disability or age will influence the process. The nurse can help by recognising the losses that patients and families may face.

Loss of role	Loss of identity	Loss of life
Loss of dreams and aspirations	Loss of a genetic legacy	Loss of self-worth
Loss of a future	Loss of body image	Loss of a relationship
Loss of faith	Loss of hope	Loss of dignity

Loss evokes a range of emotional, physical and behavioural responses.

Reflection

Consider a time when you have lost something very important. What did you feel? At the time and then afterwards.

You may be able to identify with the following responses: disbelief, denial, anger with yourself/others, fear, anxiety, sadness, regret, shame. Response to LOSS is GRIEF.

The role of the nurse is to help adjust to these losses as they can prove to be barriers to adjustment. This can be done by supporting DISTRESS (emotional, existential – concerning life and death – spiritual).

Adjustment

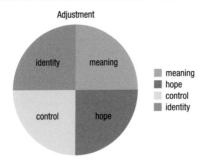

- meaning
- hope
- control
- identity

■ FINDING MEANING

1 Making sense of the illness. *'Why me?' 'I'm too young to die'*
   - You won't know the answers – there may be no answers
   - But you can listen
   - Seek spiritual support
   - Look at the value of their life (see below)
2 It also involves making sense of one's life. Mary Vachon describes it as *'taking time to look back on one's life, looking to the future and what might have been, and learning to live in the present'*
   - Talk about the patient/family's lives through stories, photos, memories. Leaving a legacy to be remembered by. A legacy box with important items. Writing letters.

Reference / Vachon, M. (2003) Emotional problems of the patient in palliative medicine. In Doyle, D., Hanks, G., Cherney, N. and Calman, K. (eds) *Oxford Handbook of Palliative Medicine* 3rd edition. USA: Oxford University Press.

Fostering hope
Described as *'to believe in one's ability to have control over one's circumstances' 'that something positive will happen'* – enabling choice, shared decision making. Not removing hope.

Restoring control
Information giving, choice, respecting autonomy. Managing symptoms.

Preserving identity
Attention to detail, body image, sexuality – privacy and intimacy.

Spiritual care
Spiritual care is about getting to the essence of the person. Who they are?
- It may be expressed through religion
- It's everyone's responsibility not just chaplaincy
- It concerns communication and relationship
- It concerns searching for meaning and purpose
- It means understanding personal belief systems and how they differ
- It means knowing how we can make it happen

Summary
- Living in the last few months of life is often within the context of uncertainty. *How much time do I have? How well will I be?*
- Emotions can be barriers or facilitators to adjustment
- The nurse may find his/her role challenged and developed as he/she looks for creative and meaningful ways to support

> *'Life will go on without me I will just miss it so'*
> Ruth Picardie

Care in the last few weeks, days, hours

Often seen as changing gear

Key aims
- Enabling a good death
- Care priorities change – comfort, minimising distress
- Supporting family and carers

Bear in mind
- In the final weeks and days it may seem as if the patient begins to disengage
- It is a time for endings and goodbyes
- Some patients and families may experience fear and anxiety, others peace and acceptance
- Care decisions may need to be made by patients, families and carers, e.g. stopping treatments, not starting treatments
- Patients and families may be weary

Reflection

What would be your good death?

This might include being pain free, being able to say goodbye, making peace with God, dying with others around you, dying alone.

At this moment of the patient's journey it is hoped that their understanding of what is a good death would be understood by others.

■ LIVERPOOL CARE PATHWAY

The Liverpool Care Pathway is a template to guide the delivery of care to the dying to complement the skill and expertise of the practitioner.

Aims

- To improve the quality of care of the dying in the last hours/days of life
- Initial assessment, ongoing assessment and care after death
- Key domains – physical, psychological, social and spiritual

Assessment

The multiprofessional team have agreed the patient is dying and at least two of the following criteria apply:

- The patient is bed-bound
- Semi-comatose
- Only able to take sips of fluid
- No longer able to take tablets

Key aspects of the pathway

- Symptom control – pain, nausea, etc. Use of continuous subcutaneous infusion (CSCI) via syringe driver to administer medication if appropriate
- Comfort measures – pressure areas, mouth care, etc.
- Anticipatory prescribing of medication
- Discontinuation of inappropriate interventions
- Psychological and spiritual care
- Care of the family (before and after death)

PATIENT NEED	AIM OF CARE	INTERVENTION
Pain free	• To identify when patient in pain if they are not able to say • Ensure pain management is comprehensive	• Assess non-verbal cues • Ensure that analgesia continues as prescribed • Using parenteral routes, set up syringe driver. Oral morphine converted to S/C morphine or morphine or diamorphine CSCI via syringe driver • PRN medications • Anticipatory prescribing and just in case box for home use

PATIENT NEED	AIM OF CARE	INTERVENTION
Receive essential patient care to maintain comfort	• Maintain comfort	• Use pressure relieving mattress • Reposition for comfort only • Assess skin integrity
Avoid unnecessary interventions	• Discontinue unnecessary medical interventions • Ensure patient and family understand • To deliver care that reflects patients ACP • Document or LPA decisions	• DNAR • S/C fluids may continue but would not be commenced at this stage. IV fluids should be discontinued • Discontinue antibiotics • Reduce BM testing • Deactivate ICDs • Stop other interventions, e.g. NIPPV
Maintain dignity	• Care respects the individual and is person centred • Empower and promote choice and control	• Privacy • Involve in decision making • Sensitive communication • Integrity of identity • Inclusion and enabling relationships
Peace or as they would wish to be	• Ensure that spiritual needs have been met	• Contact relevant spiritual advisor • Respect religious and cultural preferences

PATIENT NEED	AIM OF CARE	INTERVENTION
Say goodbye	• Ensure that there are opportunities to say goodbye	• Ensure privacy • Know how and when relatives can be contacted
Terminal agitation (An acute delirium, manifesting as a restless agitation during the terminal phase)	• Enable rest/ peace	• Provide considerable support for patient and family – explain • Use midazolam, or levomepromazine (Nozinan) CSCI via syringe driver • Ensure there is no other symptom control problem left untreated, e.g. urinary retention, spiritual distress • Remain with patient (if patient has requested not to be alone) • Ensure room is not in shadow, maintain low light • Music • Gentle hand massage, e.g. 'M' technique

PATIENT NEED	AIM OF CARE	INTERVENTION
Respiratory tract secretions	• Minimise the death rattle • Distress for family	• Explain to family • Drugs will not 'dry up' secretions already present • Treatment should be started as soon as symptoms appear Hyoscine hydrobromide start 1.2 mg CSCI via a syringe driver over 24 hours or use Glycopyrronium or Hyoscine Butylbromide
Prevent vomiting/ nausea	• Prevent vomiting • Promote fresh mouth	• Cyclizine s/c or CSCI via a syringe driver up to a maximum dose of 150 mgs in 24 hours or Haloperidol or Levomepromazine
Breathlessness	• Minimise breathlessness	• Morphine • Midazolam

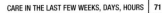

■ MOUTH CARE: AIM TO PROMOTE COMFORT

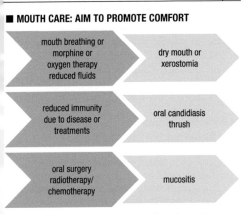

mouth breathing or morphine or oxygen therapy reduced fluids	dry mouth or xerostomia
reduced immunity due to disease or treatments	oral candidiasis thrush
oral surgery radiotherapy/ chemotherapy	mucositis

- A thorough assessment – voice, swallow, taste, lips, tongue, saliva, mucous membranes, gums, teeth, dentures, pain, smell
- Use a small-headed soft–medium toothbrush
- Fluoride toothpaste
- Clean tongue from back to front
- Clean lips with warm water. Moisten with KY jelly or oral balance gel
- Remove dentures at night and clean
- Mouthwashes include: warm saline, chlorhexidine gluconate

Treatment for oral candidiasis
- Nystatin
- Soak dentures and toothbrushes in sodium hypochlorite (Milton)

Treatment for dry mouth

- Water, ice cubes
- Saliva stimulants if patient well enough, e.g. chewing gum
- Artificial saliva, e.g. Saliva Orthana

Action

Read your local policy concerning CSCI/syringe driver.

■ RECOGNISING DEATH

- As the body becomes less active, the demand for oxygen is reduced to a minimum
- Occasionally in last few hours of life breathing gives a noisy rattle, due to a build up of mucus in the chest – medication may reduce this, as may careful change of position. It seems that this noisy breathing is not distressing to the patient
- Colour changes to the skin
- Cold to the touch
- Breathing pattern may change again with shallow, irregular breaths. There may be long pauses between breaths
- Gradually there will be longer pauses between each breath until the last one is taken (often the last breath might be 2–3 minutes from the penultimate one)

■ CARE AFTER DEATH

Action

Read local policy and refer to Guidance for Staff Responsible for Care After Death National End of Life Programme 2011.

Summary
- Care in the last few days requires preparation to enable a good death
- The Liverpool Care Pathway is one way to facilitate this

*'How someone dies lives on in the memory
of those left behind.'*
Dame Cicely Saunders

Supporting family and carers

Serious illness affects families in terms of relationships, roles and responsibilities. Families may begin grieving before the death has occurred.

Your role
- Enable privacy
- Communicate openly, honestly and regularly
- Enable opportunities for intimacy (embarrassment may prevent the asking)
- Facilitate opportunities or places for rest?
- Provide information about processes, e.g. post death
- Families may be grieving: provide opportunities to talk about how they feel, what they may fear
- Liaise with others in the team: chaplaincy for spiritual support, social worker for financial advice or support with children, doctors for information about patient's condition
- Know who to contact for post bereavement support, collect resources
- Understand cultural differences, the importance of religious or cultural beliefs or ritual and how you can make it happen

Bereavement

Bereavement support may be limited in acute or community settings. Grief may manifest in a number of ways depending on relationship, age and culture.

Action
Read about theories of loss, grief and bereavement

Understanding a family's circumstances may make you more aware of what support may be needed. This includes the social support available, if they are young/old or ill themselves, the nature of the illness and the dying. Some of these factors may put them at risk during bereavement.

Summary
- Palliative care is about supporting families along the patient journey. The quality of that support will differ depending on where care is delivered
- Grief may start before death
- This is a multiprofessional responsibility

Looking after self

- Know your support networks and their roles
- Understand your coping strategies good and bad. Try to have more good than bad!
- Recognise signs of stress in yourself
- Take up clinical supervision if it is offered, if not find a buddy
- Use reflective practice as a means to let off steam, or catharsis

- Equip yourself with the right knowledge and skills
- Develop assertiveness and managing challenging emotional situations
- Talk about it

Maybe this section should have come at the beginning of the book!

Useful websites

Information about the Gold Standards Framework
www.goldstandardsframework.org.uk

Information about the Liverpool Care Pathways
www.mcpcil.org.uk

An open learning site – education resources for caring for cancer patients
www.cancernursing.org

Information about the National End of Life Care Programme Initiatives
www.endoflifecareforadults.nhs.uk